COMPLETE GUIDE TO MALABSORPTION SYNDROME

The Comprehensive Resource To Understanding, Diagnosing, Managing Digestive Health, Symptoms, Causes, Treatment, And Nutrition Strategies

DEHART HAIRSTON

© [DEHART HAIRSTON], [2024]

All rights reserved. No part of this publication may be reproduced, distributed, or transmitted in any form or by any means, including photocopying, recording, or other electronic or mechanical methods, without the prior written permission of the publisher, except in the case of brief quotations embodied in critical reviews and certain other noncommercial uses permitted by copyright law.

DISCLAIMER

This book's content is only intended for general informative purposes. At the time of writing, the author has taken every precaution to guarantee that the material is correct and current. Nevertheless, the author disclaims all explicit and implicit representations and guarantees about the availability, appropriateness, correctness, completeness, and usefulness of the material on these pages.

Since the author is not a licensed medical practitioner, the material in this book shouldn't be interpreted as medical advice. Before making any modifications to their diet, exercise regimen, or medical treatment, readers are urged to speak with a licensed healthcare provider.

Moreover, the author has no connection to any of the businesses, organizations, or people that are discussed in this book. Any mentions of goods, services, businesses, or people are purely informative and do not indicate endorsement or suggestion.

This book's content is entirely dependent on the author's expertise, study, and comprehension of the topic. Despite having taken reasonable care to offer correct information, the author disclaims all liability for any mistakes or omissions in the material as well as for any losses, harm, or damages resulting from using the information.

It is recommended that readers use their own judgment and discretion when applying the knowledge in this book to their own situations. The use or implementation of any material in this book may result in unfavorable repercussions, directly or indirectly, for which the author assumes no liability.

By reading this book, you agree to release and hold the author harmless from any claims, losses, liabilities, costs, or expenditures resulting from or related to the use of the information you get from it.

Table of Contents

CHAPTER 1 13
- Understanding Malabsorption Syndrome 13
- What Is Malabsorption Syndrome? 13
- Causes Of Malabsorption Syndrome 14
- Common Symptoms 16
  - 1. Diarrhea: 16
  - 2. Weight Loss: 16
  - 3. Bloating and cramping in the abdomen: 16
  - 4. Exhaustion and Weakness: 17
  - 6. Alterations in the Skin, Hair, and Nails: 17
  - 7. Anemia: 18
  - 8. Unexpected Bleeding or Bruising: 18

CHAPTER 2 19
- Digestive System Overview 19
- How The Digestive System Works 19
- Role Of Enzymes And Hormones 20
- Absorption Process 21

CHAPTER 3 25
- Types Of Malabsorption 25
- Different Types Of Malabsorption 25

Celiac Disease 25
Lactose Intolerance 27
Tropical Sprue..28
CHAPTER 4 31
Diagnostic Tools 31
Blood Tests 31
Stool Tests 33
Imaging Techniques 36
CHAPTER 5 39
Treatment Options 39
Dietary Changes 39
Vitamin And Mineral Supplements...............41
Medications 42
Surgery (If Necessary) 44
CHAPTER 6 47
Managing Symptoms 47
Coping With Digestive Discomfort................47
Lifestyle Modifications...................................50
Providing Supportive Treatments 52
CHAPTER 7 57
Complications And Risks 57

Nutritional Deficiencies 57
Bone Health Issues 59
Other Health Complications 61

CHAPTER 8 63
Diet And Nutrition 63
Recommended Foods For Malabsorption 63
Foods To Avoid 64
Meal Planning Tips 66

CHAPTER 9 69
Living With Malabsorption 69
Practical Tips For Daily Life 69
   1. Dietary Modifications: 69
   2. Enzyme Replacement Therapy: 70
   3. Nutritional Supplements: 70
   4. Hydration: 70
   5. Smaller, More Often Meals: 71
   6. Stress Management: 71
   7. Frequent Exercise: 72
   8. Medication Management: 72
   9. Symptom Monitoring: 72
   10. Frequent Follow-Up: 73

Social And Emotional Support 73

    1. Join Support Groups: 74

    2. Inform Loved Ones: 74

    3. Seek Professional Assistance: 74

    4. Exercise Self-Care: 75

    5. Be Upfront About Your Requirements: 75

    6. Keep in Touch: 75

    8. Seek Balance: 76

    9. Have patience with yourself: 77

Maintaining A Positive Outlook 77

    2. Realistic Goal-Setting: 78

    3. Practice thankfulness: 78

    4. Remain Informed: 78

    5. Discover Happiness in Ordinary Times: 79

    6. Engage in Mindfulness Practices: 79

    7. Seek Support: 79

    8. Emphasis on Self-Care: 80

    9. Remain Adaptable: 80

    10. Celebrate Your Strength: 81

CHAPTER 10 83

Prevention And Future Outlook 83

Preventing Malabsorption Syndrome 83
Research And Developments 86
Looking Ahead: Living A Healthy Life 88
CONCLUSION 92
THE END 95

ABOUT THE BOOK

"Malabsorption Syndrome" is a thorough manual that provides priceless insights into a disorder that affects millions of people worldwide. It is more than simply a book. Answers to questions that people struggling with malabsorption need may be found within its pages.

The trip starts with Chapter 1, which introduces readers to the fundamentals of malabsorption syndrome, dissecting its intricacies and illuminating its causes and signs. It's important to comprehend the condition, and this chapter provides the framework for the remainder of the book.

Next, Chapter 2 delves further into the complex operations of the digestive system for readers. Here, students discover the crucial functions that hormones, enzymes, and the absorption process itself play.

With this understanding, readers will be more able to understand the next chapters, which explore the many kinds of malabsorption, ranging from Lactose Intolerance and Tropical Sprue to Celiac Disease.

A ray of hope appears in Chapter 4, which lists the diagnostic techniques used by medical experts to determine if a patient has malabsorption. Readers learn about the processes required for a correct diagnosis, from blood testing to imaging methods, which sets the stage for the efficient treatment approaches covered in Chapter 5.

However, "Malabsorption Syndrome" goes beyond diagnosis and therapy, touching on symptom management in Chapter 6. Readers get useful advice on how to adjust their lifestyle, accept supporting treatments, and deal with intestinal pain.

Furthermore, Chapter 7 of the book addresses the dangers and difficulties of malabsorption head-on, highlighting the need to be watchful to preserve general health. To provide a comprehensive approach to controlling the disease, chapters 8 and 9 include advice on food and nutrition in addition to useful recommendations for everyday life and emotional support.

In summary, Chapter 10 provides readers with the necessary information to avoid malabsorption syndrome and provides an overview of current research and advances. It also summarizes the preventative strategy and perspective for the future.

To put it simply, "Malabsorption Syndrome" is a lifeline for anyone navigating the intricacies of this ailment, not just a book. It is an invaluable resource for patients, caregivers, and healthcare professionals alike because of its thorough coverage and helpful guidance.

CHAPTER 1

Understanding Malabsorption Syndrome

What Is Malabsorption Syndrome?

A collection of conditions known as malabsorption syndrome occurs when the body is unable to adequately absorb nutrients from the food you eat. These nutrients, which are necessary for the body to operate normally, include proteins, lipids, carbs, vitamins, and minerals. Due to shortages in these essential nutrients, poor absorption may result in several health issues.

The intricate network that breaks down food absorbs nutrients, and gets rid of waste is called the digestive system. The majority of nutritional absorption takes place in the small intestine, therefore problems there often cause malabsorption syndrome, which impairs this process. Malabsorption may be caused by diseases including

Crohn's disease, pancreatic insufficiency, and celiac disease that damage the lining of the intestines or decrease the synthesis of digestive enzymes.

Causes Of Malabsorption Syndrome

Malabsorption syndrome may arise from a variety of causes, including lifestyle choices, underlying medical disorders, and genetic predispositions. Damage to the lining of the small intestine, which may be brought on by infections, celiac disease, or inflammatory bowel disease (IBD), is one of the main causes.

The autoimmune condition known as celiac disease is brought on by eating gluten and causes damage to the lining of the small intestine, which impairs nutritional absorption. Similar to this, Crohn's disease, another kind of IBD, impedes nutrition absorption by causing ulcers and inflammation in the digestive system.

Another prevalent cause of malabsorption is pancreatic insufficiency. The digestive enzymes required for food digestion in the gut are produced by the pancreas. Appropriate digestion and absorption are hampered when the pancreas is unable to create adequate enzymes, as is the case with diseases like pancreatic cancer and chronic pancreatitis.

Furthermore, the structure of the digestive system might change as a result of some surgical operations, such as gastric bypass surgery, which can impact nutritional absorption. Malabsorption syndrome may result from bacterial overgrowth in the small intestine, which can also impede nutrient absorption. This disease is known as small intestinal bacterial overgrowth (SIBO).

Common Symptoms

Early diagnosis and treatment of malabsorption syndrome depend heavily on the ability to recognize its symptoms. Common symptoms include the following, however, they might vary according to the underlying reason and the nutrients that are lacking.

1. **Diarrhea:** Prolonged diarrhea is a classic sign of malabsorption, meaning the body is not taking in enough nutrients. Fat that hasn't been digested might make stool thick, oily, and smell bad.

2. **Weight Loss:** Even with a regular diet, inadequate nutrition absorption might cause unintentional weight loss. This is especially apparent when there is significant malabsorption.

3. **Bloating and cramping in the abdomen:** People who are malabsorbing may bloat, cramp, and feel uncomfortable in their abdomen, usually after

eating. The buildup of undigested food in the intestines may be the cause of this.

4. Exhaustion and Weakness: Deficiencies in some nutrients, particularly those about vitamins and minerals such as calcium, iron, and B vitamins, may cause exhaustion, weakness, and a general decrease in energy levels.

5. Deficiencies in some nutrients might cause symptoms that are specific to them. For example, a low calcium level might result in muscular cramps and bone discomfort, while a vitamin B12 deficiency can induce neurological symptoms like tingling in the hands and feet.

6. Alterations in the Skin, Hair, and Nails: The state of the skin, hair, and nails might be impacted by the malabsorption of certain vitamins and minerals.

For instance, a zinc deficit may cause brittle nails and hair loss, while a vitamin A shortage might cause dry, rough skin.

7. Anemia: Fatigue, weakness, and pallor are some of the symptoms of anemia, which is caused by a decreased body's ability to absorb iron, folate, or vitamin B12.

8. Unexpected Bleeding or Bruising: Vitamin K deficiency, which is vital for blood clotting, may cause profuse bleeding and easy bruises.

Diagnosing these symptoms may be difficult because of their variability in intensity and potential for comorbidity with other gastrointestinal illnesses. Therefore, if you encounter chronic or worrisome symptoms of malabsorption syndrome, it's imperative that you see a healthcare provider for the correct diagnosis and treatment.

CHAPTER 2

Digestive System Overview

How The Digestive System Works

The digestive system is a biological engineering wonder that masterfully coordinates a myriad of procedures to convert food into nutrients the body can use. Carbohydrate digestion starts in the mouth with chewing and salivation. Food next passes down the esophagus and into the stomach, where enzymes and stomach acids further break down proteins and eradicate dangerous microorganisms.

The bulk of nutritional absorption takes place in the small intestine, where the partly digested meal next goes. Here, the liver's bile and the pancreas' specialized enzymes help break down lipids, proteins, and carbs into their most basic forms. Villi and microvilli, which are microscopic projections that resemble fingers and line the inside of the small intestine, enhance the surface area available for absorption.

Ultimately, undigested food and waste materials pass into the large intestine, where they are converted into stool and eliminated by the rectum and anus. This is also where water and electrolytes are absorbed.

Role Of Enzymes And Hormones

Hormones and enzymes are essential to the digestive process because they make sure that food is absorbed and broken down properly. Enzymes break down complicated compounds into simpler forms that the body can absorb. They are biological catalysts that accelerate chemical processes. For instance, lipases break down lipids, proteases break down proteins, and amylase breaks down carbs.

Conversely, hormones control the release of enzymes and the passage of food through the digestive system, among other elements of digestion. For example, cholecystokinin causes the release of pancreatic enzymes and bile, while gastrin increases the production of stomach acid.

Enzymes and hormones work in tandem to maintain a well-regulated and synchronized digestive system that enables the body to absorb the nutrients it needs from meals and flush out waste.

Absorption Process

The small intestine is the main site of absorption, where nutrients are absorbed by the body and used for several physiological processes. Enterocytes are specialized cells that line the inside of the small intestine. They have different transport pathways that let them absorb nutrients more easily.

Glucose is produced during the breakdown of carbohydrates and is taken up by enterocytes via certain transporter proteins. Similar to this, certain transporters are used to absorb fatty acids from lipids and amino acids from proteins.

These nutrients are either promptly used by the enterocytes for energy or are transferred into the circulation and distributed to all of the body's cells. While fat-soluble nutrients like vitamins A, D, E, and K are absorbed into the lymphatic system before entering the circulation, water-soluble nutrients like glucose and amino acids reach the bloodstream immediately.

Nutrients that enter the large intestine unabsorbed in the small intestine are either fermented by microorganisms or eliminated as waste.

Comprehending the complex functions of the digestive system, encompassing the functions of enzymes and hormones, along with the process of absorption, is essential for an understanding of malabsorption disorders and their impact on the body's capacity to absorb nutrients from meals.

CHAPTER 3

Types Of Malabsorption

Different Types Of Malabsorption

A variety of disorders where the small intestine is unable to effectively absorb nutrients are together referred to as malabsorption syndrome. For diagnosis and therapy, knowledge of the various forms of malabsorption is essential. Let's examine the three main categories: Tropical Sprue, Lactose Intolerance, and Celiac Disease.

Celiac Disease

An autoimmune condition called celiac disease is brought on by eating gluten. In those with celiac disease, the protein gluten—which is present in wheat, barley, and rye—damages the lining of the small intestine, impairing nutritional absorption. There is a broad range of symptoms that might include non-gastrointestinal symptoms like exhaustion, anemia, and even neurological disorders, as well as gastrointestinal symptoms including diarrhea, stomach discomfort, and bloating.

A combination of blood tests to look for certain antibodies and an intestinal biopsy to confirm small intestine damage are used to diagnose celiac disease. The mainstay of treatment is rigorous adherence to a gluten-free diet. Intestinal healing and successful symptom management may result from removing gluten from the diet.

Being gluten intolerant necessitates being cautious while reading food labels and preventing cross-contamination. Fortunately, there are more gluten-free options accessible due to increased awareness of gluten sensitivity, which makes it simpler for people with celiac disease to maintain a balanced diet.

Lactose Intolerance

A widespread illness known as lactose intolerance is caused by low amounts of the enzyme lactase, which prevents the body from breaking down lactose, the sugar present in milk and dairy products. Insufficient lactase causes lactose to enter the colon undigested, resulting in symptoms including gas, diarrhea, bloating, and pain in the abdomen.

A lactose tolerance test or a hydrogen breath test, in which high hydrogen levels in the breath after lactose consumption suggest malabsorption, are often used to diagnose lactose intolerance. The mainstay of treatment is dietary changes, such as cutting less on lactose or supplementing with lactase enzymes to help with digestion.

Thankfully, there are many of lactose-free substitutes out now, such as lactose-free yogurt, cheese, and milk, which makes it simpler for those who are lactose intolerant to enjoy dairy products without experiencing any pain.

Tropical Sprue

Malabsorption disorders such as tropical sprue mainly afflict people who travel to or reside in tropical climates, including the Caribbean, South Asia, and Latin America. Although the precise etiology of tropical sprue is unknown, it is thought to be the consequence of parasite or bacterial infections that harm the small intestine's lining and impede the body's ability to absorb nutrients.

Tropical sprue may cause exhaustion, diarrhea, weight loss, and vitamin and mineral deficits. Diagnosis entails using stool testing, intestinal biopsies, and blood tests to rule out other causes of malabsorption. Antibiotics are usually prescribed to treat any underlying illnesses, and vitamin and mineral supplements are used to make up for any deficiencies.

Keeping oneself clean, avoiding contaminated food and drink in endemic areas, and practicing excellent hygiene are all important ways to prevent tropical sprue. Even though tropical sprue may be crippling if ignored, a complete recovery is possible with early diagnosis and adequate care.

Healthcare providers must be aware of these many forms of malabsorption to properly identify and treat individuals who suffer from them. Through individualized treatment plans, people may successfully control their symptoms and enhance their overall quality of life.

CHAPTER 4

Diagnostic Tools

Blood Tests

Blood tests are essential for the diagnosis of malabsorption syndromes and provide important information about a number of the condition's features. These tests evaluate many factors, including the function of critical organs involved in digestion and absorption, inflammatory indicators, and nutritional levels. Since malabsorption often results in deficits in these vital nutrients, blood tests to detect levels of vitamins, minerals, and proteins are among the most typically conducted.

Due to the gastrointestinal tract's poor absorption of essential nutrients, vitamin and mineral deficits are frequent in malabsorption disorders. Low levels of minerals like calcium and iron, as well as vitamins like folate, vitamin D, and vitamin B12, may be found by blood testing. These deficits might show up in a range of symptoms, from weakness and exhaustion to neurological issues and bone abnormalities.

Additionally, blood tests may identify anomalies in protein levels, such as hypoalbuminemia, which indicates excessive loss or poor absorption of proteins. A vital protein produced by the liver, albumin is essential for balancing bodily fluids and moving different chemicals throughout the circulation. Low albumin levels may indicate additional gastrointestinal illnesses or underlying malabsorption problems.

Furthermore, inflammatory indicators that might indicate the existence of inflammation in the body, such as erythrocyte sedimentation rate (ESR) and C-reactive protein (CRP), may be evaluated by blood tests.

Inflammatory bowel disease (IBD) and celiac disease are two malabsorption diseases that are often linked to persistent inflammation in the gastrointestinal system.

In conclusion, blood tests are essential for the diagnosis of malabsorption disorders because they may identify inflammatory indicators, aberrant protein levels, and nutritional deficits. These examinations direct future diagnostic and therapeutic approaches and provide insightful information about the fundamental reasons for malabsorption.

Stool Tests

Stool tests—also referred to as stool exams or fecal analyses—are crucial diagnostic instruments for determining the presence of malabsorption disorders. To assess several elements of gastrointestinal health, such as digestion, absorption, and microbial balance, these tests analyze the content of stool samples.

The amount of fat in stools is one of the main things that is tested. Steatorrhea, or the presence of extra fat in the feces, is a disorder caused by malabsorption syndromes, which often result in decreased fat digestion and absorption. A common sign of malabsorption illnesses including pancreatic insufficiency and celiac disease is diarrhea, which results in oily, bulky, and odorous feces.

Additionally, undigested food particles might be an indicator of insufficient digestion and absorption in the gastrointestinal system and are evaluated for in stool tests. Stool samples may also include undigested proteins and carbs in addition to lipids, which might provide light on the degree of malabsorption.

Additionally, anomalies in fecal enzymes involved in the digestion of proteins and lipids, such as chymotrypsin and elastase, may be identified by stool testing. Decreases in these enzyme levels might be a sign of pancreatic insufficiency, a disorder that impairs the absorption of nutrients due to insufficient pancreatic production of digesting enzymes.

Additionally, stool tests could look for infections, parasites, or microbial imbalances in the gut, all of which can aggravate gastrointestinal symptoms and malabsorption. Determining the underlying cause of malabsorption and directing suitable treatment techniques may be facilitated by identifying such organisms or dysbiosis.

To sum up, stool tests are useful diagnostic instruments that evaluate lipid content, undigested food particles, fecal enzymes, and the microbial balance in the gastrointestinal system to identify malabsorption disorders. These examinations provide medical professionals with crucial data for correctly detecting and treating malabsorption diseases.

Imaging Techniques

Because they allow for the visualization of the gastrointestinal tract's anatomy and function, imaging methods are essential for the diagnosis of malabsorption disorders. The non-invasive imaging technologies provide significant insights into potential causes of malabsorption, such as motility problems, mucosal inflammation, and structural abnormalities.

Abdominal ultrasonography, which creates comprehensive pictures of the liver, gallbladder, pancreas, and intestines using high-frequency sound waves, is one of the most widely used imaging methods.

Gallstones, pancreatic cysts, and intestinal strictures—all of which may impede digestion and absorption—can be seen by ultrasound.

Computed tomography (CT) scanning is another imaging technique used in the diagnosis of malabsorption. CT scanning creates cross-sectional pictures of the belly and pelvis using X-rays. With the use of CT scans, anomalies like tumors, inflammation, or abscesses that may impair gastrointestinal function may be found. These scans also offer extensive information on the density and structure of the abdominal organs.

Additionally, malabsorption disorders are evaluated using magnetic resonance imaging (MRI), which is especially useful for evaluating soft tissue structures and vascular anomalies in the belly. For individuals with suspected malabsorption, MRI is a safe and useful imaging method since it offers good contrast resolution and doesn't use ionizing radiation.

To evaluate intestinal motility and transit time, functional imaging tests such as small bowel follow-through and enteroclysis may be carried out in addition to these anatomical imaging methods. In these tests, contrast chemicals are consumed or infused, and then serial imaging is used to monitor the flow of contrast through the small intestine. This helps to detect anatomical abnormalities or motility issues that may be linked to malabsorption.

In conclusion, imaging methods are useful diagnostic instruments for assessing malabsorption syndromes because they allow the visualization of gastrointestinal tract motility issues, mucosal inflammation, and structural anomalies. These imaging methods provide doctors with the crucial information they need to properly diagnose and treat malabsorption problems.

CHAPTER 5

Treatment Options

Dietary Changes

Changing one's diet is essential for treating malabsorption syndrome. Optimizing nutrition absorption while reducing intestinal discomfort is the main objective. One of the most important tactics is to modify the diet to fit the unique requirements of the person, which often entails cutting down on or removing certain food kinds that make symptoms worse.

A low-FODMAP diet, which limits fermentable carbohydrates that may cause gastrointestinal symptoms including gas, bloating, and diarrhea, is a popular strategy. Foods rich in fermentable sugars, such as some fruits, vegetables, cereals, and dairy products, must be avoided while following this diet. People with malabsorption syndrome may enhance nutrient absorption and reduce digestive pain by consuming less of these poorly absorbed carbs.

Including foods that are simple to digest in the diet may also help reduce symptoms and guarantee that enough nutrients are consumed. To facilitate digestion and lessen the strain on the gastrointestinal system, this may include eating smaller, more frequent meals. Furthermore, as cooked or processed meals are often simpler for the body to break down than raw or fibrous ones, choosing them may help with digestion and absorption.

Meal time and portion sizes are crucial considerations in addition to changing the kinds of meals ingested. Eating three big meals a day might overburden the digestive system and improve nutritional absorption. Instead, eat smaller meals throughout the day.

To prevent overburdening the intestines and aggravating symptoms, portion management is also crucial.

Vitamin And Mineral Supplements

To correct dietary imbalances caused by malabsorption syndrome, supplementation is often required since the condition may result in deficits in important vitamins and minerals. Physicians may prescribe different supplements to restore depleted nutrients based on the particular deficits found by blood testing or other diagnostic procedures.

For malabsorption syndrome, vitamin B12, vitamin D, iron, calcium, and magnesium supplements are often recommended. These nutrients are essential for the production of red blood cells, healthy bones, and healthy muscles, among other physiological activities. Individuals with malabsorption syndrome may avoid or lessen symptoms related to deficiencies and promote general health and well-being by taking supplements of these vitamins and minerals.

It's crucial to remember that supplementation has to be customized to meet the specific requirements of each person and properly monitored by a medical practitioner. Doses of certain vitamins and minerals should be carefully adjusted depending on parameters such as age, sex, weight, and underlying health issues, since excessive consumption of these nutrients may cause toxicity and bad consequences.

Medications

Medication may sometimes be recommended to treat malabsorption syndrome patients' symptoms and enhance intestinal health. Depending on the underlying cause of malabsorption, these drugs try to relieve certain symptoms such as diarrhea, stomach discomfort, inflammation, or bacterial overgrowth.

For instance, to manage diarrhea and minimize fluid loss, doctors may prescribe anti-diarrhea drugs like loperamide. H2-receptor antagonists and proton pump inhibitors (PPIs) may lessen the production of stomach acid, which may assist with acid reflux or peptic ulcer symptoms that are often linked to malabsorption syndrome.

Antibiotics may also be recommended to address small intestinal bacterial overgrowth, which may worsen symptoms by interfering with the absorption of nutrients. Antibiotics may aid in restoring the balance of the gut microbiota and enhancing digestive function by specifically targeting and eradicating harmful bacteria.

Surgery (If Necessary)

Surgery may be thought of as a last option in severe instances of malabsorption syndrome that does not respond to conservative therapy methods. Usually, problems such as intestinal blockage, strictures, fistulas, or other anatomical abnormalities that produce severe gastrointestinal symptoms or limit the absorption of nutrients are saved until surgery.

Depending on the underlying cause and degree of intestinal damage, common surgical therapies for malabsorption syndrome include intestinal resection, strictureplasty, or intestine bypass surgery. With these procedures, damaged sections of the intestine are removed or bypassed, normal intestinal architecture is restored, and digestion and nutritional absorption are enhanced.

It is crucial to remember that not every person with malabsorption syndrome needs or benefits from surgery, and this should only be considered as a last resort after all other treatment options have been exhausted. To balance the potential risks and advantages and guarantee the best possible result for the patient, the decision to have surgery should be made in collaboration with a multidisciplinary healthcare team that includes gastroenterologists, surgeons, dietitians, and other experts.

CHAPTER 6

Managing Symptoms

Coping With Digestive Discomfort

Although managing malabsorption syndrome-related gastrointestinal distress may be difficult, there are several techniques you can use to reduce symptoms and enhance your quality of life. Finding the foods that make your symptoms worse is one of the first stages. Maintaining a diet journal may be quite beneficial in identifying certain foods that can be problematic. Once these triggers have been recognized, you may decrease pain by reducing or eliminating their intake.

Paying attention to your eating habits is another essential component of managing stomach pain. Smaller, more frequent meals spread out throughout the day may help your digestive system function more smoothly and improve nutritional absorption. To facilitate digestion and lessen the chance of bloating and pain, chew your meal well and eat slowly. Preventing the escalation of symptoms may also be achieved by avoiding heavy, oily foods and big meals.

Certain lifestyle modifications, in addition to food modifications, may also have a major impact on the management of digestive pain. Frequent physical activity might enhance digestive health by inducing bowel motions and mitigating abdominal distension. Stress may significantly affect gastrointestinal function, thus practicing stress management strategies like yoga, meditation, or deep breathing exercises might help reduce symptoms brought on by or made worse by stress.

Additionally, maintaining enough hydration is essential for promoting healthy digestion and nutritional absorption. Try to stay hydrated during the day by drinking plenty of water and minimizing your consumption of liquids that might exacerbate symptoms, such as alcohol or caffeinated drinks. When ingested in moderation, herbal drinks such as ginger or peppermint tea may help soothe the digestive tract and ease pain.

If dietary and lifestyle changes are made but the pain in the stomach does not go away, it could be required to use over-the-counter or prescription medicine to properly control symptoms. Antacids may assist in balancing stomach acid and relieve heartburn or indigestion, while drugs such as laxatives or antidiarrheals can treat constipation or diarrhea brought on by malabsorption syndrome. To make sure a new pharmaceutical regimen is safe and suitable for your particular condition, you must speak with a healthcare provider before beginning it.

Lifestyle Modifications

Changing one's lifestyle is often essential to controlling symptoms related to malabsorption syndrome. You may assist your digestive system and enhance your general health by making certain adjustments. Changing to a nutrient-dense diet that emphasizes foods high in vitamins, minerals, and other necessary nutrients is one of the most significant lifestyle changes you can make. Despite possible problems with malabsorption, you can make sure you're receiving the nutrients your body needs by including plenty of fruits, vegetables, lean meats, whole grains, and healthy fats in your meals.

Stressing the importance of gut health and encouraging a healthy microbiota is another crucial lifestyle change. Eating foods high in probiotics, such as kefir, kimchi, sauerkraut, and yogurt, may help your gut become more colonized with good bacteria, which can aid in digestion and absorption of nutrients. Furthermore, prebiotic foods like onions, garlic, bananas, and asparagus help feed these good bacteria and maintain a healthy gut environment.

In addition, regular exercise is crucial for controlling the symptoms of malabsorption syndrome. Exercise may enhance digestive health by encouraging bowel motions, boosting circulation, and lowering stress. To get the most out of your physical activity, try to include cardiovascular, strength, and flexibility workouts.

Furthermore, to promote general health and well-being, it is important to give priority to rest and sleep. Your body, especially your digestive system, can heal and rebuild when you get enough sleep each night. Developing a soothing nighttime ritual, adhering to a regular sleep schedule, and maintaining proper sleep hygiene may all help you get better sleep and feel less stressed, which may assist with stomach issues.

Finally, reducing exposure to certain triggers or irritants may aid in preventing flare-ups of symptoms. This might include giving up alcohol, quitting smoking, and avoiding foods and drinks that you know make your symptoms worse. Malabsorption syndrome may be efficiently managed and your quality of life enhanced by deliberate lifestyle alterations.

Providing Supportive Treatments

Supportive therapy, in addition to dietary and lifestyle adjustments, may be very important in treating the symptoms of malabsorption syndrome. To enhance overall results, these therapies are intended to be used in conjunction with conventional medical treatments to target certain components of the problem.

Supplementing with nutrients is a popular supportive treatment used to treat malabsorption syndrome. Supplementing may help close nutritional gaps and avoid deficits since people with this illness may have trouble absorbing certain nutrients from meals. Healthcare providers may prescribe supplements, such as vitamin B12, iron, calcium, vitamin D, and fat-soluble vitamins A, D, E, and K, depending on each patient's unique requirements and deficits.

Enzyme replacement therapy is another supportive treatment that may be helpful in the management of malabsorption syndrome. Supplemental digestive enzymes are taken as part of this treatment to aid in the breakdown of proteins, lipids, and carbohydrates in the digestive system and improve nutritional absorption. Malabsorption syndrome is often caused by pancreatic insufficiency, which is usually treated with pancreatic enzyme replacement therapy.

In addition, complementary and alternative treatments like chiropractic adjustments, herbal remedies, and acupuncture may provide further assistance in treating digestive issues and enhancing general health. Although more studies are necessary to completely comprehend the effectiveness of these treatments for malabsorption syndrome in particular, some patients find them beneficial when used in conjunction with other forms of comprehensive care.

Furthermore, because having a chronic illness may hurt mental health, psychological assistance can be quite helpful for those with malabsorption syndrome. Individuals may improve resilience and quality of life by learning coping mechanisms and navigating the emotional difficulties related to their disease with the use of counseling, support groups, and mindfulness-based treatments.

All things considered, supportive therapies serve as a valuable supplement to traditional medical care and enable people with malabsorption syndrome to actively participate in their health management. Despite the difficulties caused by malabsorption syndrome, patients may maximize their results and enhance their general well-being by including these treatments in a thorough treatment plan.

CHAPTER 7

Complications And Risks

Nutritional Deficiencies

Numerous dietary deficits resulting from malabsorption syndrome may have a substantial negative influence on one's general health and well-being. The body may become deficient in certain vitamins, minerals, proteins, and lipids when vital nutrients are not efficiently absorbed.

A typical feature of malabsorption syndrome is vitamin deficits. Since fat-soluble vitamins like A, D, E, and K need to be properly absorbed to be used, they are especially impacted. Vitamin A deficiency may cause immune system weakness and visual issues. Low levels of vitamin D have been linked to problems with bone health, including osteoporosis and a higher risk of fractures.

A vitamin K shortage may result in irregular bleeding and poor blood clotting, while a vitamin E deficiency can induce muscular weakness and nerve damage.

Mineral shortages are also common, particularly when iron, calcium, magnesium, and zinc absorption is hampered by malabsorption. Anemia from iron deficiency may cause weariness, weakness, and pallor. Both osteoporosis and bone demineralization are influenced by calcium shortage. Weakness, irregular pulse, and cramping in the muscles may result from a magnesium deficit. Lack of zinc has an impact on a child's development, immune system, and ability to heal wounds.

Malabsorption of fat and protein may cause immunological dysfunction, weight loss, muscular atrophy, and deficits in vital fatty acids. It can also aggravate skin and hair issues.

All things considered, the nutritional inadequacies associated with malabsorption syndrome highlight the need for focused treatments to address particular nutrient shortages and promote general health.

Bone Health Issues

Malabsorption syndrome has a major effect on bone health because it causes shortages in important minerals that are necessary for the construction, mineralization, and strength of bones, such as calcium, vitamin D, vitamin K, and magnesium.

The main building block of bone tissue is calcium, and a lack of it may result in lower bone density and an increased risk of osteoporosis and fractures. The metabolism of bones and the absorption of calcium depends heavily on vitamin D. A vitamin D deficiency may hinder the absorption of calcium, further weakening bones and raising the risk of fracture.

The production of proteins involved in bone mineralization requires vitamin K. Its absence might hinder the growth of new bones and raise the possibility of fractures. Due to its role in bone mineralization and regulation of calcium metabolism, magnesium is also essential for the health of bones.

Impaired absorption of these nutrients exacerbates problems with bone health in malabsorption syndrome, increasing the risk of fractures, osteopenia, and osteoporosis. Thus, maintaining bone health and avoiding problems connected to bones requires treating dietary deficiencies and making sure enough calcium, vitamin D, vitamin K, and magnesium are consumed.

Other Health Complications

Malabsorption syndrome may result in several other health problems affecting different organ systems in addition to dietary inadequacies and problems with the health of the bones.

Consequences of decreased absorption of carbs, lipids, and other nutrients might include diarrhea, gas, bloating, and stomach discomfort. Dehydration, electrolyte imbalances, and dietary deficits may worsen the symptoms of chronic diarrhea.

Steatorrhea, which is characterized by greasy, rancid feces because of an excess of fat in the stool, may be caused by malabsorption of lipids. This not only hurts but also suggests that the body is not absorbing enough of the important fatty acids, which may lead to immune system impairment and skin issues.

Moreover, malabsorption syndrome may have an impact on the pancreas, liver, and gallbladder, which can result in issues including gallstones, pancreatitis, and liver dysfunction. To properly treat these issues, which further exacerbate digestive symptoms, specialized therapies could be necessary.

Furthermore, if left untreated, malabsorption syndrome may hurt a child's general growth and development, including delayed growth, failure to thrive, and developmental delays.

Malabsorption syndrome is a systemic disorder that requires comprehensive management strategies to address its multifaceted effects. Individuals with the disorder are also more likely to develop nutritional-related conditions like anemia, neuropathy, and immune system dysfunction.

CHAPTER 8

Diet And Nutrition

Recommended Foods For Malabsorption

It's critical to prioritize readily digested, nutrient-dense meals for managing malabsorption syndrome. Lean meats, fish, eggs, and tofu are examples of readily digested proteins that may provide needed amino acids without overtaxing the digestive system. The absorption of fat-soluble vitamins may be facilitated by including foods high in healthy fats, such as avocados, nuts, and seeds.

Consuming a diet rich in fruits and vegetables is crucial if you want to receive your fill of fiber, vitamins, and minerals. Some raw veggies, meanwhile, could be difficult for people to digest if they have problems with malabsorption. Vegetables may be kinder to the digestive system and yet contain important nutrients when they are cooked or steamed.

Whole grains that don't upset your stomach, such as quinoa, rice, and oats, maybe a wonderful source of fiber and carbs. Furthermore, foods that have undergone fermentation, such as kefir, sauerkraut, and yogurt, contain healthy microorganisms that help enhance digestion and promote gut health.

Foods To Avoid

Certain foods should be restricted or avoided completely since they may worsen the symptoms of malabsorption. Foods that are high in fat, fried, or highly processed might be difficult for the digestive system to break down, which can exacerbate symptoms like diarrhea and discomfort in the abdomen.

People with lactose intolerance, a frequent condition linked to malabsorption syndrome, may find it difficult to digest dairy products. To help with digestion, it is best to use lactase enzyme supplements or choose lactose-free dairy alternatives.

Certain people with malabsorption problems may experience gas and bloating while eating foods high in fiber, such as beans, lentils, and cruciferous vegetables. Although fiber is necessary for a healthy digestive system, it may be advantageous to choose low-fiber options or fully prepare these meals to facilitate simpler digestion.

Foods that are very hot or acidic might aggravate the gastrointestinal system and make symptoms like indigestion and heartburn worse. Steer clear of spicy spices and sauces, as well as acidic fruits like citrus and tomatoes, since they may assist ease malabsorption-related pain.

Meal Planning Tips

Malabsorption syndrome sufferers may control their symptoms and make sure they're receiving enough nutrients by organizing their meals well. To start lightening the load on the digestive system and avoid overloading the colon, start by breaking meals into smaller, more frequent amounts.

To guarantee that your intake of vitamins, minerals, and macronutrients is balanced, concentrate on including a range of nutrient-rich meals in each meal. Try diverse cooking techniques, such as baking, grilling, or steaming, to increase food digestibility without sacrificing nutritious content.

You can discover triggers and make educated decisions about what to include in your diet by maintaining a food diary to note how various foods impact your symptoms. Personalized advice and assistance in creating a meal plan customized to your requirements and tastes may also be obtained by consulting with a licensed dietitian.

Make being hydrated a priority by consuming plenty of water throughout the day. being properly hydrated is crucial for promoting healthy digestion and nutrition absorption. Preventing dehydration and reducing gastrointestinal discomfort may also be achieved by limiting alcohol and caffeine intake.

Individuals with malabsorption syndrome may successfully manage their symptoms and maintain appropriate nutrition for general health and well-being by adhering to these suggestions and implementing helpful meal-planning strategies.

CHAPTER 9

Living With Malabsorption

Practical Tips For Daily Life

Although having malabsorption syndrome might bring particular difficulties in day-to-day living, there are doable ways to control symptoms and enhance general health.

1. Dietary Modifications: Changing one's diet is an important part of treating malabsorption. This entails identifying meals that are simpler to absorb and digest by working closely with a dietician or healthcare provider. This can include swapping out high-fat or high-fiber meals that are known to aggravate symptoms for easier-to-digest alternatives like lean meats, cooked veggies, and refined grains.

2. Enzyme Replacement Therapy: People who have malabsorption may find that this treatment is helpful in some circumstances. This is adding extra enzymes to meals to aid in digestion and enhance the absorption of nutrients. Depending on the underlying cause of malabsorption, these enzymes might include bile acid supplements, lactase, or pancreatic enzymes.

3. Nutritional Supplements: Taking nutritional supplements may be recommended to guarantee appropriate intake of key vitamins and minerals, since malabsorption syndrome may result in nutrient shortages. Depending on the inadequacies found in your blood tests and your particular requirements, your healthcare practitioner could suggest certain supplements.

4. Hydration: If diarrhea is not well treated, it may result in dehydration. Diarrhea is a typical sign of malabsorption.

It's critical to maintain proper hydration throughout the day by consuming plenty of liquids, such as clear broths, electrolyte-rich drinks, and water. It's also advised to stay away from alcohol and caffeine since these might make dehydration worse.

5. Smaller, More Often Meals: Throughout the day, eating smaller, more often meals might help reduce the discomfort that malabsorption-related digestive issues can cause. This may lessen the strain on the digestive system and lower the possibility of overfeeding the body with big meals, which might make symptoms worse.

6. Stress Management: For those who have malabsorption syndrome, stress might make their digestive problems worse. Developing appropriate coping mechanisms for stress, such as mindfulness meditation, relaxation exercises, or fun hobbies, may enhance general well-being and lessen the negative effects of stress on digestive health.

7. Frequent Exercise: For those with malabsorption syndrome, regular exercise might aid with digestion and general health. To boost general well-being, lower stress levels, and encourage digestive motility, combine aerobic, strength, and flexibility workouts.

8. Medication Management: It's critical to adhere to your healthcare provider's medication management instructions if malabsorption is brought on by an underlying illness, such as Crohn's disease or celiac disease. This might include using drugs to treat underlying illnesses, inhibit the immune system, or control inflammation.

9. Symptom Monitoring: By keeping a record of your symptoms, you can spot trends and situations that might make your malabsorption worse. Keep track of your eating habits, emotional state, and any digestive symptoms you encounter throughout the day in a symptom journal.

Together with your healthcare professional, you may use this knowledge to make well-informed choices regarding treatment and dietary changes.

10. Frequent Follow-Up: It's important to schedule routine follow-up visits with your healthcare practitioner to keep an eye on your condition, make any treatment adjustments, and address any new or worsening symptoms. Make an effort to notify your healthcare team of any concerns or changes in your symptoms, as well as to schedule follow-up consultations.

Social And Emotional Support

Living with malabsorption syndrome may affect one's social and emotional as well as physical health. It is crucial to look for assistance from loved ones, friends, and medical specialists to manage the difficulties associated with this disease.

1. **Join Support Groups:** Making connections with other people who have malabsorption syndrome may be very beneficial in terms of understanding and support. Joining a support group, whether in person or virtually, may help you share stories, get advice on how to manage symptoms, and get emotional support from others who understand your challenges.

2. **Inform Loved Ones:** Sharing information about malabsorption syndrome and its effects on everyday life with your friends and family might be beneficial. By doing so, they will be better able to comprehend your requirements and, if needed, provide assistance and accommodations.

3. **Seek Professional Assistance:** Don't be afraid to contact a therapist or counselor if you need assistance with the emotional effects of malabsorption syndrome. Therapy may provide a secure environment in which you can examine your

emotions, create coping mechanisms, and discover practical approaches to stress and anxiety management.

4. Exercise Self-Care: Taking care of your mental health is equally as vital as your physical health. Schedule time for enjoyable self-care activities, such as reading a book, going for a stroll in the outdoors, doing yoga, or engaging in a hobby.

5. Be Upfront About Your Requirements: Don't be embarrassed to let others know about your requirements and limits. Advocating for yourself is crucial to managing malabsorption syndrome, whether it is setting boundaries to safeguard your well-being, asking for assistance with meal preparation, or seeking modifications at social events.

6. Keep in Touch: Try to keep in touch with your loved ones and friends, even if it means coming up

with inventive methods to interact with them while taking care of your symptoms. Social media, phone conversations, and virtual hangouts may all help you stay in touch with people without endangering your health.

7. Even though having malabsorption syndrome might make life difficult, make an effort to keep your attention on the good things in your life. Remind yourself that you are more than your condition, celebrate your little accomplishments, and express appreciation for the things that make you happy.

8. Seek Balance: To effectively handle the mental and physical challenges of malabsorption syndrome, you must find balance in your life. Give top priority to things that feed your body and spirit, and don't be afraid to decline invitations to events that will just make your symptoms worse or deplete your vitality.

9. **Have patience with yourself:** Overcoming obstacles is a part of the process of managing malabsorption syndrome. To navigate the ups and downs of life with this disease, celebrate your resilience, be gentle with yourself, and engage in self-compassion.

Maintaining A Positive Outlook

Living with malabsorption syndrome may make it difficult to have a happy attitude, but taking charge of your life and prioritizing self-care can help you feel better overall and live a better quality of life.

1. While there may be elements of malabsorption syndrome that are out of your control, concentrate on the areas where you are in charge, such as your food, way of life, and attitude. Give yourself the ability to make decisions that will improve your health and general well-being.

2. Realistic Goal-Setting: Make sure your objectives are reasonable for you and acknowledge your accomplishments as you go. Tiny changes may have a big impact on your general health and well-being, whether it's via better nutrition, greater exercise, or better stress management.

3. Practice thankfulness: Even amid difficulties, you may change your perspective and concentrate on the good things in your life by developing a feeling of thankfulness. Every day, set aside some time to think about the blessings in your life, such as your resilient and strong self, your joyful moments, and your uplifting friends and family.

4. Remain Informed: Remain up to date on the latest advancements in therapy and management approaches as well as malabsorption syndrome. Since knowledge is power, you can successfully advocate for yourself and make educated choices about your health by equipping yourself with it.

5. Discover Happiness in Ordinary Times: Despite the difficulties associated with having malabsorption syndrome, remember to find happiness in ordinary times. Finding moments of pleasure may help elevate your spirits and enhance your attitude on life, whether it's by engaging in a pastime you're passionate about, spending time with loved ones, or indulging in a wonderful meal that goes well with your stomach.

6. Engage in Mindfulness Practices: Mindfulness practices, such as body scans, meditation, and deep breathing, may assist in lowering the tension and anxiety linked to malabsorption syndrome. Include mindfulness exercises in your everyday routine to help you unwind, elevate your mood, and develop inner peace.

7. Seek Support: When you need it, don't be afraid to ask friends, family, and medical experts for assistance.

Be in the company of a network of individuals who are sympathetic to your plight and who can provide consolation, understanding, and useful help when required.

8. Emphasis on Self-Care: Give self-care tasks that feed your body, mind, and spirit a top priority. Whether it's getting enough sleep, eating healthily, exercising often, or just spending time in nature, taking care of oneself is crucial to controlling malabsorption syndrome and keeping a happy attitude in life.

9. Remain Adaptable: Managing malabsorption syndrome may need making changes as you go along to meet new obstacles. Remain adaptable and receptive, and be prepared to explore alternative methods for treating your ailments and enhancing your standard of living.

10. Celebrate Your Strength: It takes bravery, fortitude, and strength to deal with malabsorption syndrome. Acknowledge your accomplishments on the path to improved health and well-being and celebrate your courage and fortitude in enduring the highs and lows of this illness.

CHAPTER 10

Prevention And Future Outlook

Preventing Malabsorption Syndrome

The three major strategies for preventing malabsorption syndrome include eating a balanced diet, taking care of any underlying problems, and keeping the gut healthy overall. Treating any illnesses or variables that can lead to malabsorption, such as pancreatic insufficiency, Crohn's disease, or celiac disease, is one of the most important preventative measures. Frequent visits to medical professionals may aid in the early diagnosis and treatment of many illnesses.

A healthy diet is essential for avoiding malabsorption. For the gut to work as best it can, a well-balanced diet high in nutrients—vitamins, minerals, proteins, and healthy fats—is necessary. Nutrients that assist absorption and digestion may be included in a range of fruits, vegetables, whole grains, lean proteins, and dairy products (if permitted). Malabsorption may also be avoided by limiting the amount of processed meals, sugary snacks, and high-fat foods consumed. These might cause gastrointestinal problems.

In addition, people who have malabsorption syndrome or are at risk want to think about creating a customized meal plan in collaboration with a qualified dietitian or nutritionist. Dietary adjustments, such as avoiding certain trigger foods or adding enzyme supplements to help with digestion, may be part of this approach. It's important to pay attention to your body's signals and modify your diet as necessary to relieve symptoms and enhance nutritional absorption.

Apart from eating, sustaining a healthy lifestyle may also help ward against malabsorption syndrome. Frequent exercise lowers the risk of constipation and other gastrointestinal problems by improving gut motility and stimulating digestion. By lowering inflammation and fostering a healthy gut flora, stress management practices like yoga or meditation may help improve gut health.

Last but not least, maintaining proper cleanliness and taking precautions with food will help stave against infections and gastrointestinal ailments that might worsen malabsorption. Reducing the risk of bacterial or parasite illnesses that influence gut health includes washing hands completely before handling food, cooking meats fully, avoiding intake of unpasteurized dairy products, and avoiding contaminated water.

Malabsorption syndrome may be avoided and proper gut function can be promoted by people by treating underlying causes, keeping a healthy lifestyle, choosing a nutritious diet, and practicing excellent hygiene.

Research And Developments

The fundamental causes of malabsorption syndrome are still being clarified by advances in medical research, which also open up new possibilities for diagnosis and therapy. Researchers are looking at cutting-edge diagnostic methods to pinpoint certain genetic mutations or structural anomalies that lead to malabsorption, including as genetic testing and enhanced imaging modalities.

In addition, continuing research endeavors to clarify the function of the gut microbiome in malabsorption and investigate viable measures to adjust microbial diversity and enhance gut well-being. The potential of probiotics, prebiotics, and other microbiome-targeted medicines to help people with malabsorption syndrome regain gut homeostasis and enhance their capacity to absorb nutrients is being researched.

Researchers are concentrating on understanding the effects of dietary variables on gut health and malabsorption in addition to advances in diagnosis and treatment. Recent research indicates that several food additives, gluten, and FODMAPs (fermentable oligosaccharides, disaccharides, monosaccharides, and polyols) may worsen gastrointestinal symptoms and cause malabsorption in those who are vulnerable.

Furthermore, developments in nutritional science are opening the door for the creation of specialty foods and supplements that are specifically designed to meet the dietary requirements of those who suffer from malabsorption syndrome. These items could include digestive enzymes, enhanced nutritional formulations, or other bioactive substances intended to improve nutrient absorption and reduce malabsorption symptoms.

Clinically relevant therapies for malabsorption syndrome patients need the translation of scientific findings into cooperative initiatives between researchers, healthcare practitioners, and industry partners. We can continue to increase the precision of diagnosis, hone therapeutic approaches, and eventually improve the quality of life for malabsorption patients by funding research and development projects.

Looking Ahead: Living A Healthy Life

Malabsorption syndrome patients must take proactive measures to control their symptoms, follow dietary guidelines, and regularly assess their nutritional status to lead healthy lives. Although malabsorption syndrome may be difficult to manage, people can improve their general health and well-being by making lifestyle changes and getting assistance from medical professionals.

Keeping a balanced diet that promotes adequate nutrient absorption is essential to living a healthy life with malabsorption syndrome. This might include creating a customized meal plan that takes into account each person's dietary requirements and preferences in close collaboration with a qualified dietitian or nutritionist. Reducing dietary triggers and chemicals that worsen symptoms while consuming nutrient-dense meals like fruits, vegetables, lean meats, and whole grains may help ease gastrointestinal distress and improve the absorption of vital nutrients.

For those with malabsorption syndrome, routine nutritional status monitoring is crucial in addition to dietary adjustments. This may include monitoring indicators of inadequacy or malnutrition in addition to routine blood testing to determine vitamin, mineral, and other nutrient levels. Supplementing with vitamins, minerals, or other nutrients may be advised to treat deficiencies and avoid long-term issues related to malabsorption, depending on the requirements of each person.

Furthermore, for those with malabsorption syndrome, stress management and placing a high priority on mental health may be quite important in fostering general well-being. Stress-reduction methods include deep breathing exercises, mindfulness meditation, and taking up enjoyable and relaxing hobbies and pastimes may help lower inflammation, strengthen the digestive system, and improve overall quality of life.

For those with malabsorption syndrome, keeping up a network of friends, family, and medical professionals may be a tremendous source of support. Effective management of the illness requires open discussion regarding symptoms, available treatments, and any issues or difficulties encountered along the road with healthcare practitioners.

Despite the difficulties presented by their disease, people with malabsorption syndrome may enjoy happy and healthy lives by being proactive in managing their symptoms, following dietary guidelines, placing a high priority on their mental health, and asking for help from loved ones and medical professionals. The future looks bright for those with malabsorption syndrome in terms of better outcomes and increased quality of life because of further research and developments in diagnosis and treatment.

CONCLUSION

Malabsorption syndrome is a multifactorial illness marked by the small intestine's poor absorption of nutrients, resulting in a range of nutritional deficits and gastrointestinal symptoms. We have examined its many facets throughout this investigation, taking into account its origins, symptoms, diagnosis, and available treatments.

First off, a variety of possible reasons have been found, ranging from autoimmune diseases like celiac disease to structural disorders like Crohn's disease or surgical procedures like gastric bypass. It is essential to comprehend these factors to provide precise diagnosis and focused therapy.

Second, it might be difficult to diagnose Malabsorption Syndrome since its symptoms are varied and often coexist with those of other gastrointestinal conditions.

Patients' quality of life is greatly impacted by these symptoms, which may range from persistent diarrhea and weight loss to vitamin and mineral shortages.

Thirdly, a thorough approach is needed to diagnose Malabsorption Syndrome. This includes reviewing the patient's medical history, doing a physical examination, ordering laboratory testing, doing imaging investigations, and sometimes doing invasive procedures like endoscopy or biopsy. The significance of patient-provider cooperation is emphasized by this diagnostic process.

Finally, efforts for therapy focus on managing dietary inadequacies, addressing the underlying cause, and relieving symptoms. This might include changing one's diet, taking vitamins and mineral supplements, using drugs to treat underlying illnesses or symptoms, or in extreme situations, having surgery.

Finally, it should be noted that Malabsorption Syndrome poses serious difficulties for both patients and medical professionals. Because of its varied character, diagnosis and therapy must be tailored to the individual. Furthermore, further study is necessary to improve our comprehension of its underlying processes and provide treatment strategies that work better. For those impacted by Malabsorption Syndrome, we can improve quality of life and improve outcomes by encouraging more awareness and cooperation among the medical community.

THE END

www.ingramcontent.com/pod-product-compliance
Lightning Source LLC
Chambersburg PA
CBHW070310230526
45470CB00002B/802